THE PICTURE BOOK OF
PSALMS

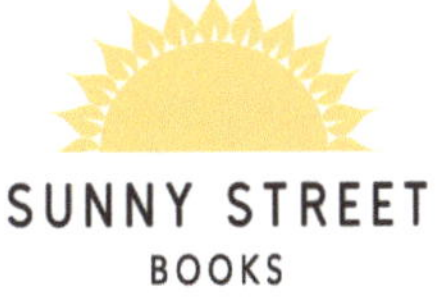

SUNNY STREET
BOOKS

The commands of the

Lord are radiant; they

give light to the eyes.

Psalm 19:8

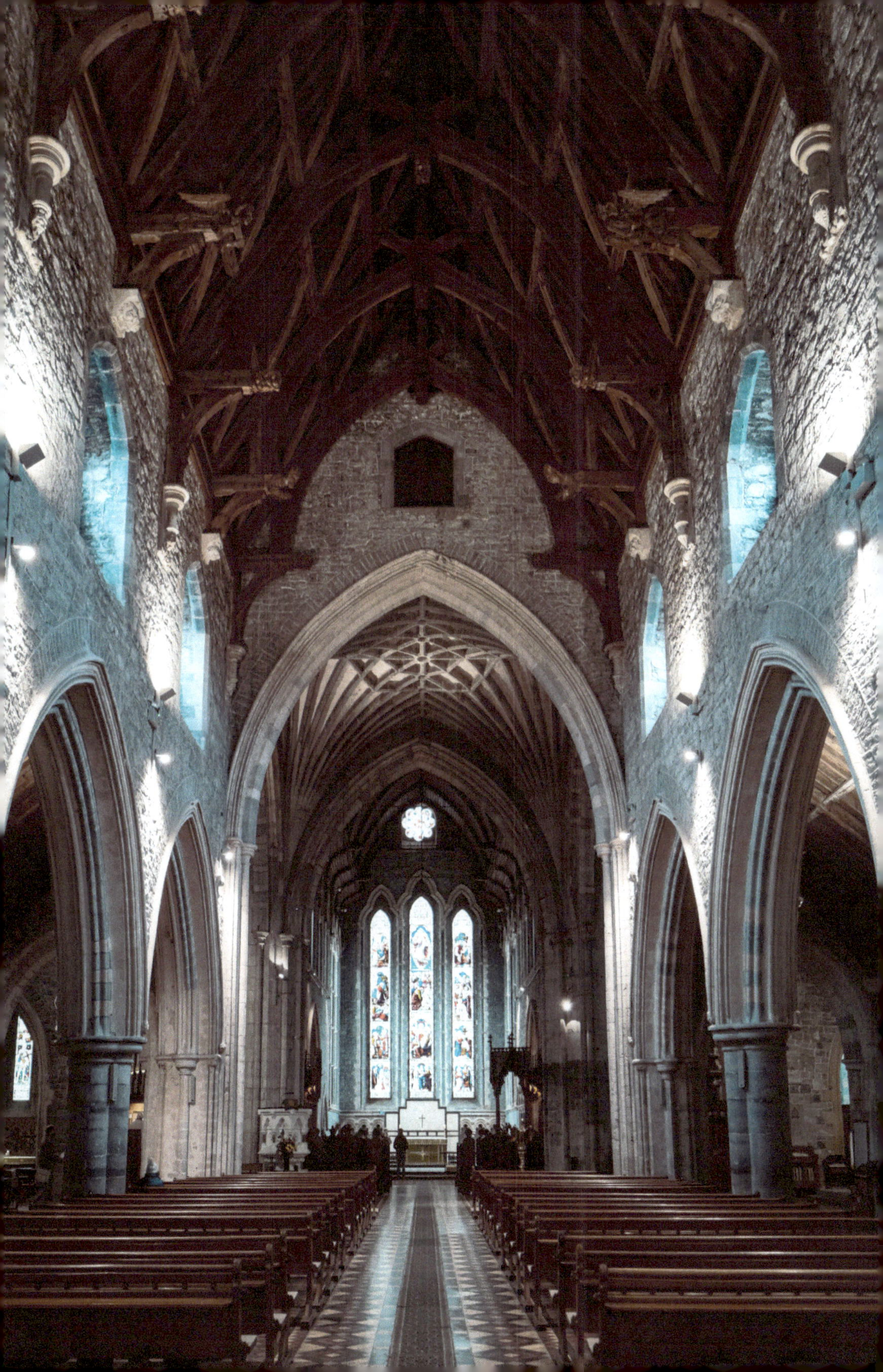

Come, let us tell of the

Lord 's greatness; let us

exalt his name together.

Psalm 34:3

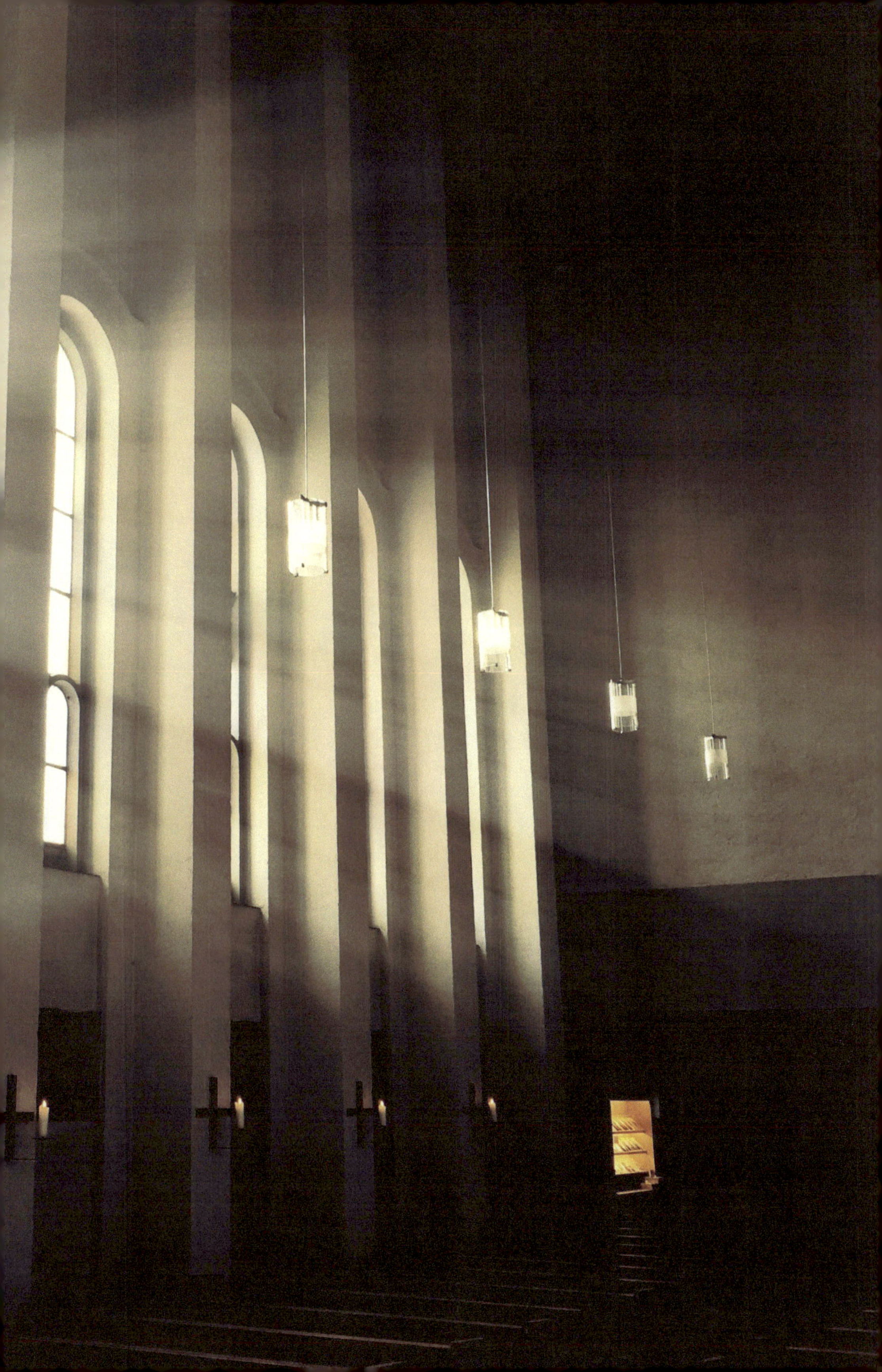

Delight yourself in

the Lord, and he will

give you the desires of

your heart.

Psalms 37:4

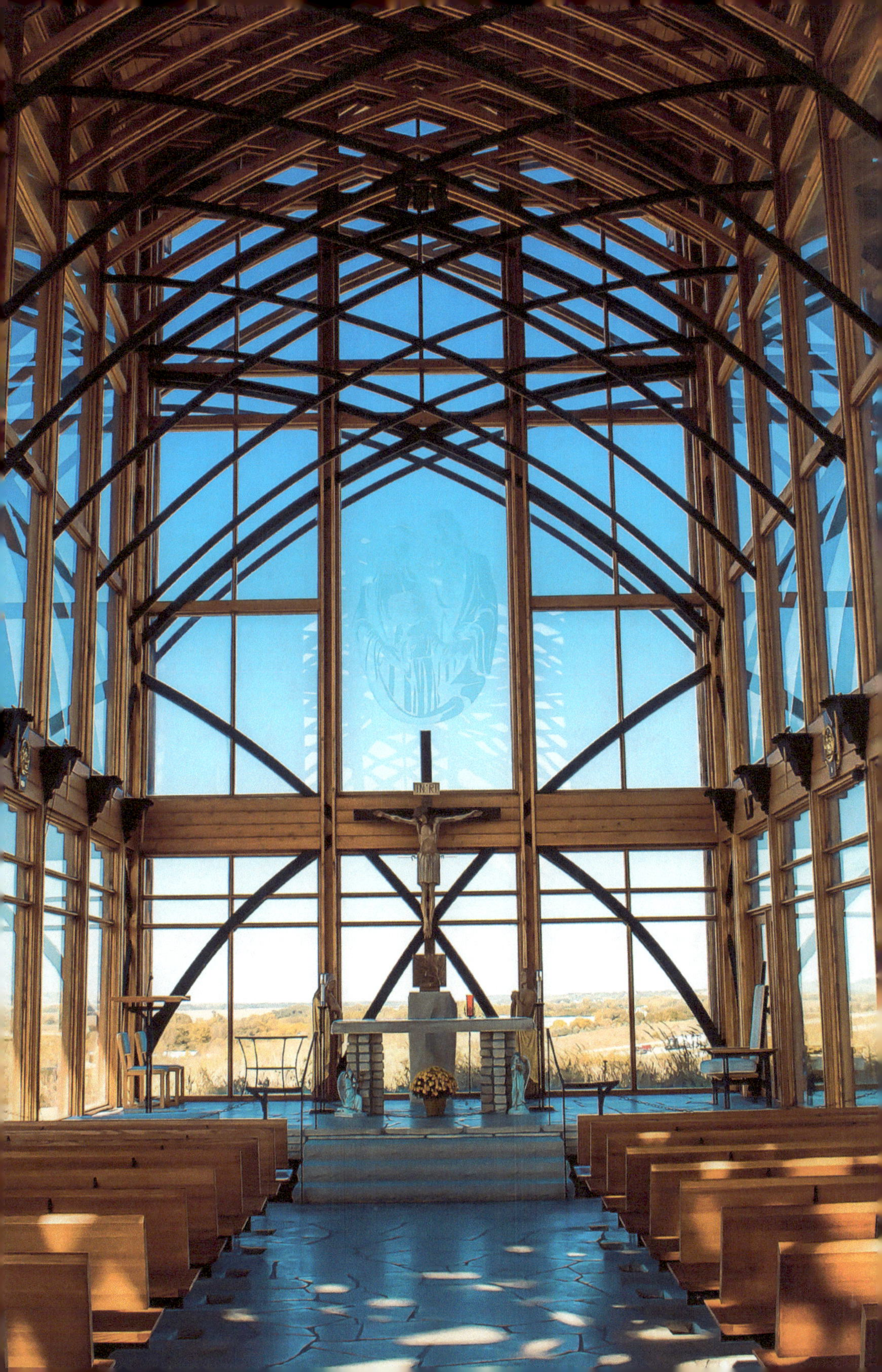

Be still and know

that I am God.

Psalm 46:10

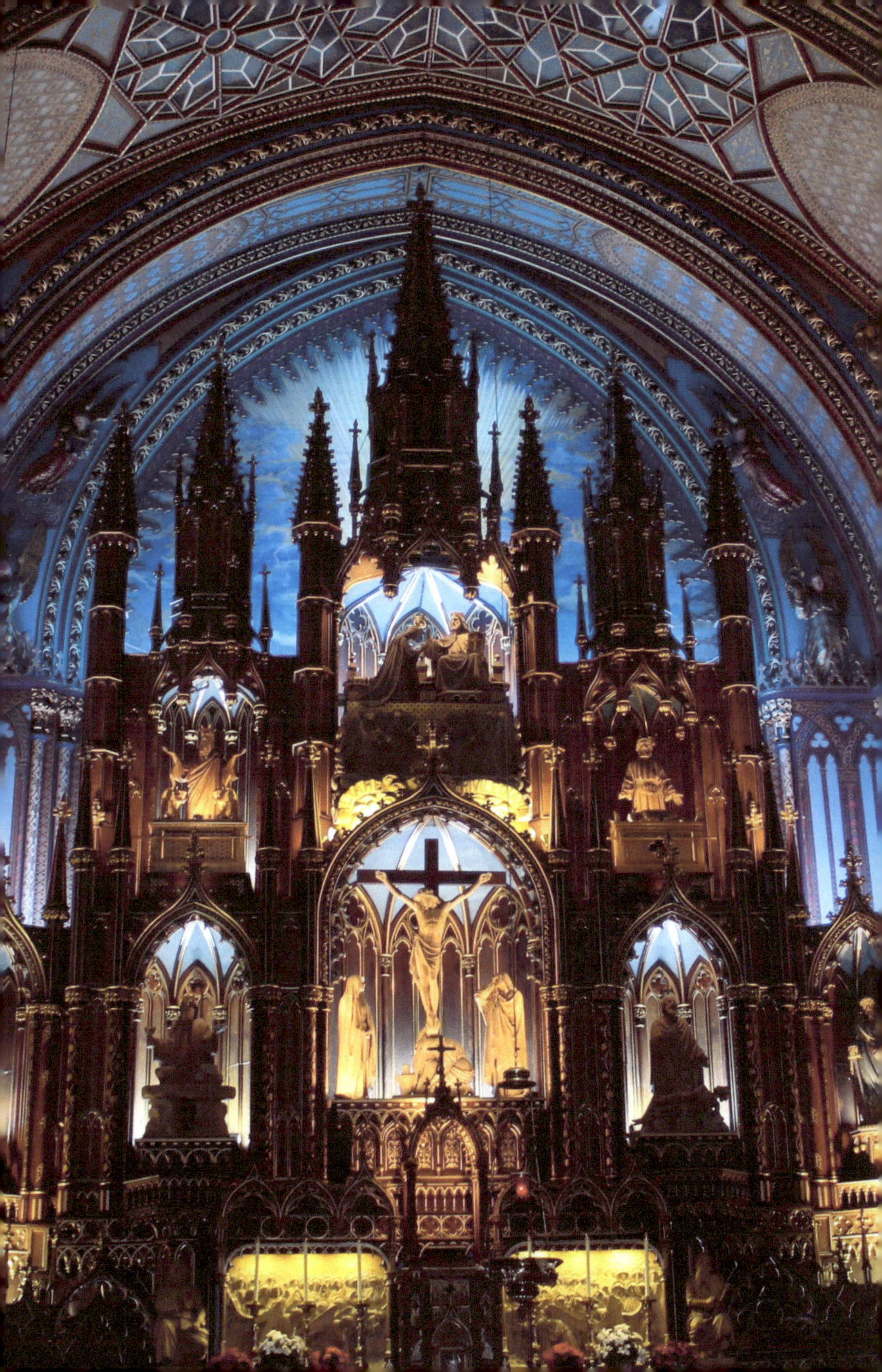

Create in me a pure

heart, O God, and renew a

steadfast spirit within me.

Psalms 51:10

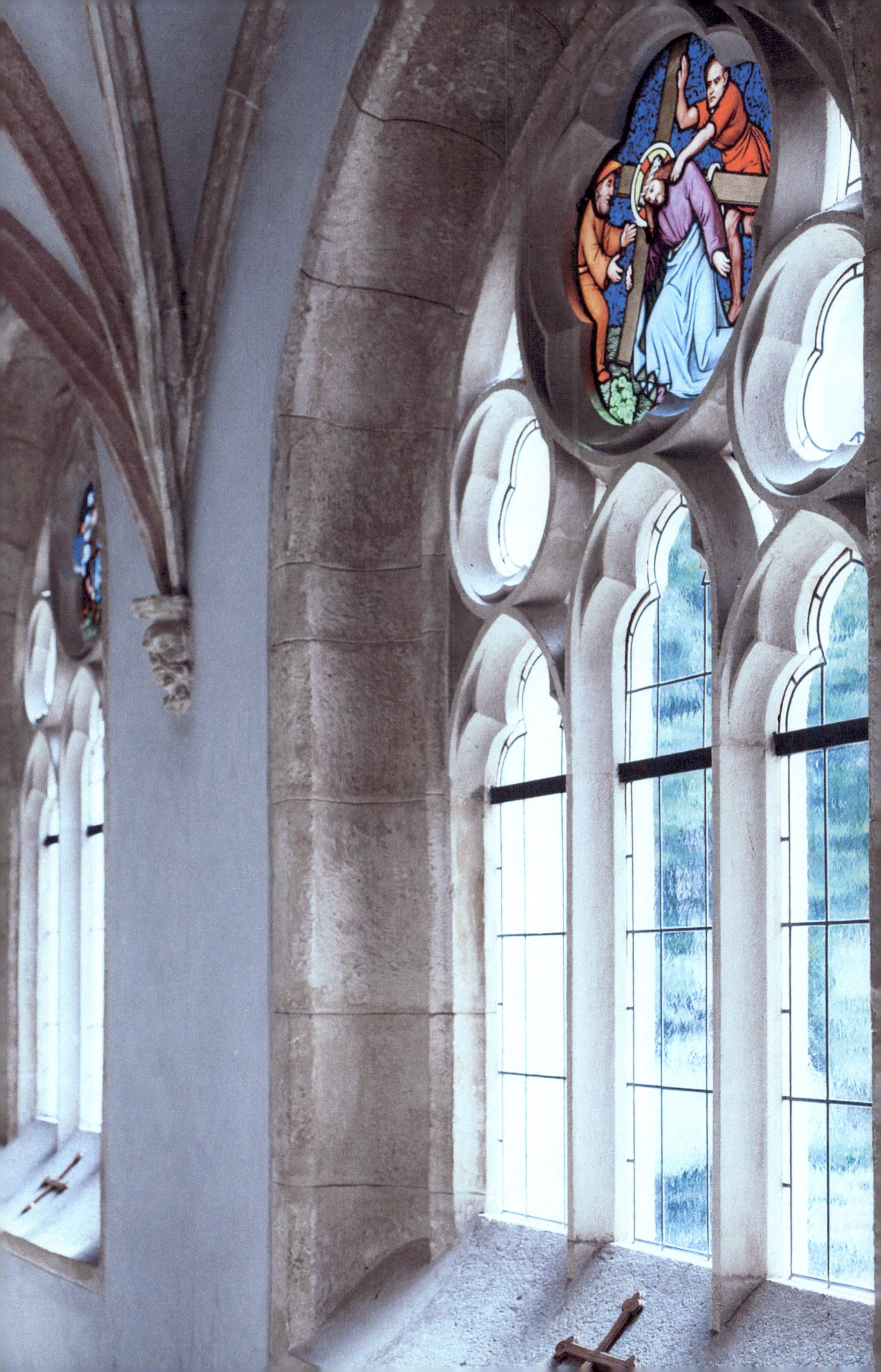

In peace I will lie

down and sleep, for you

alone, Lord, make me

dwell in safety.

Psalms 4:8

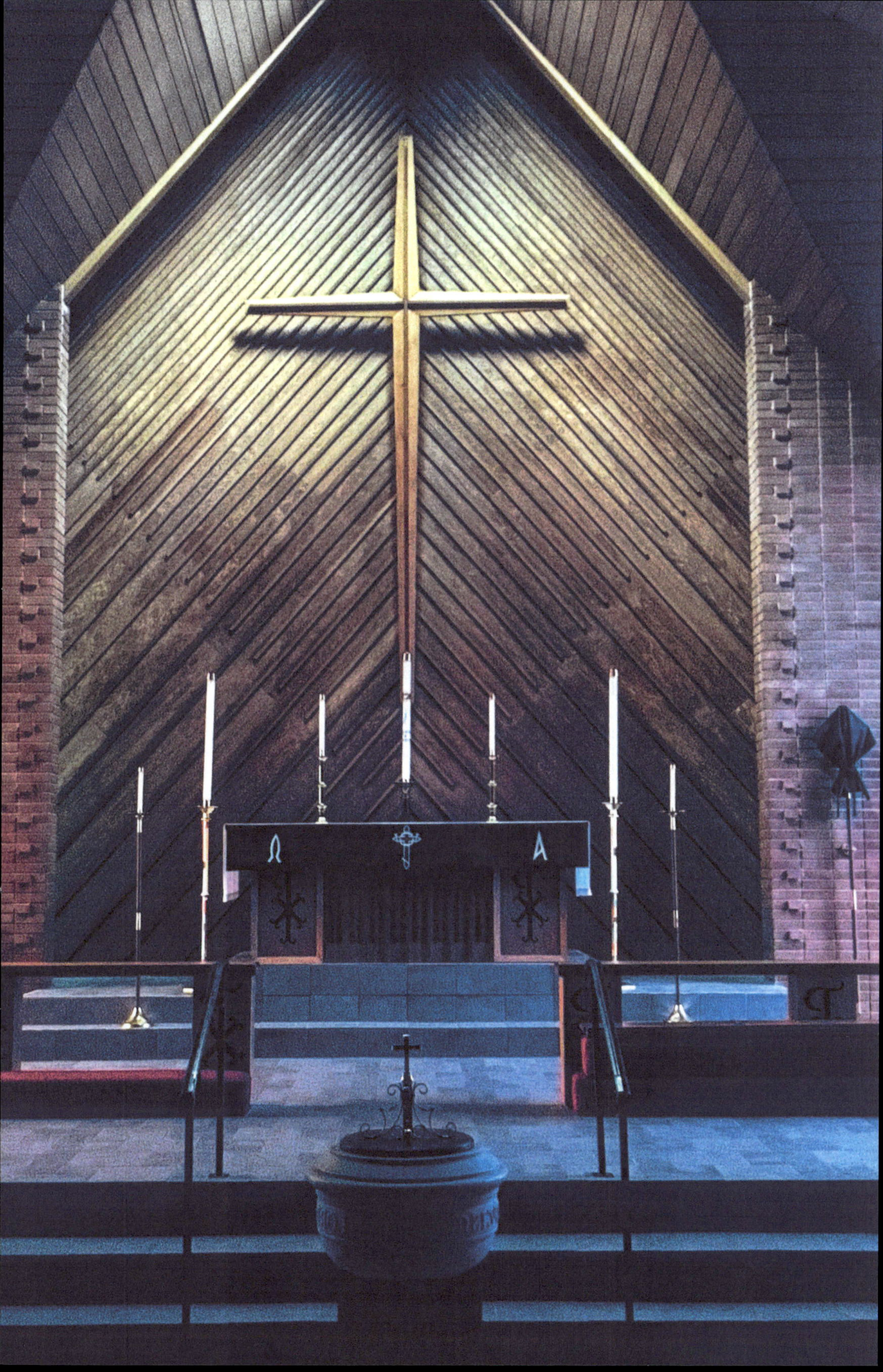

*L*ord my God,

I called to you for help,

and you healed me.

*P*salm 30:2

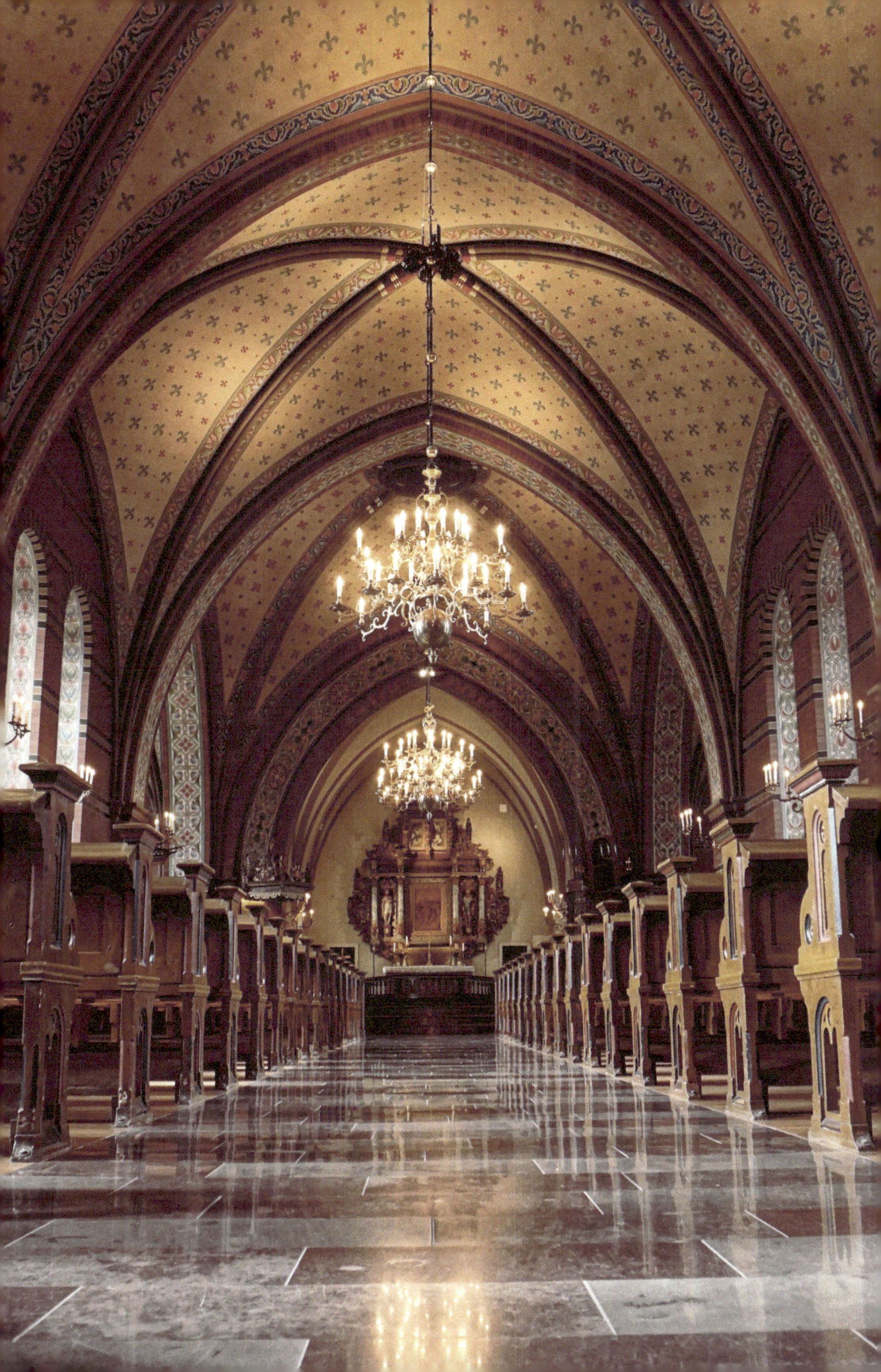

$\mathcal{W}$orship the Lord with

gladness; come before

Him with joyful songs.

$\mathcal{P}$salm 100:2

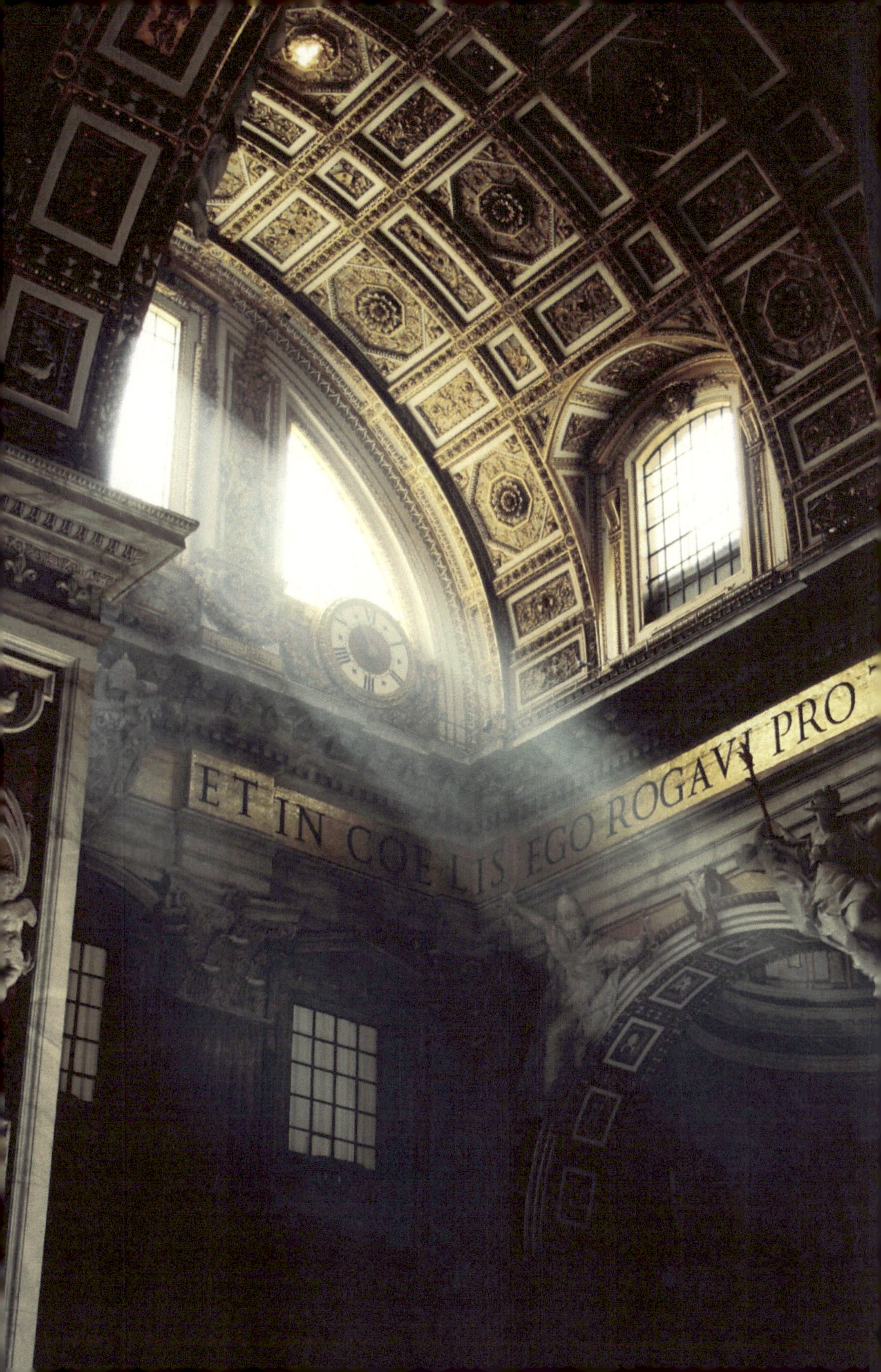
ET IN COELIS EGO ROGAVI PRO

May God be gracious

to us and bless us and

cause His face to shine

upon us.

Psalm 67:1

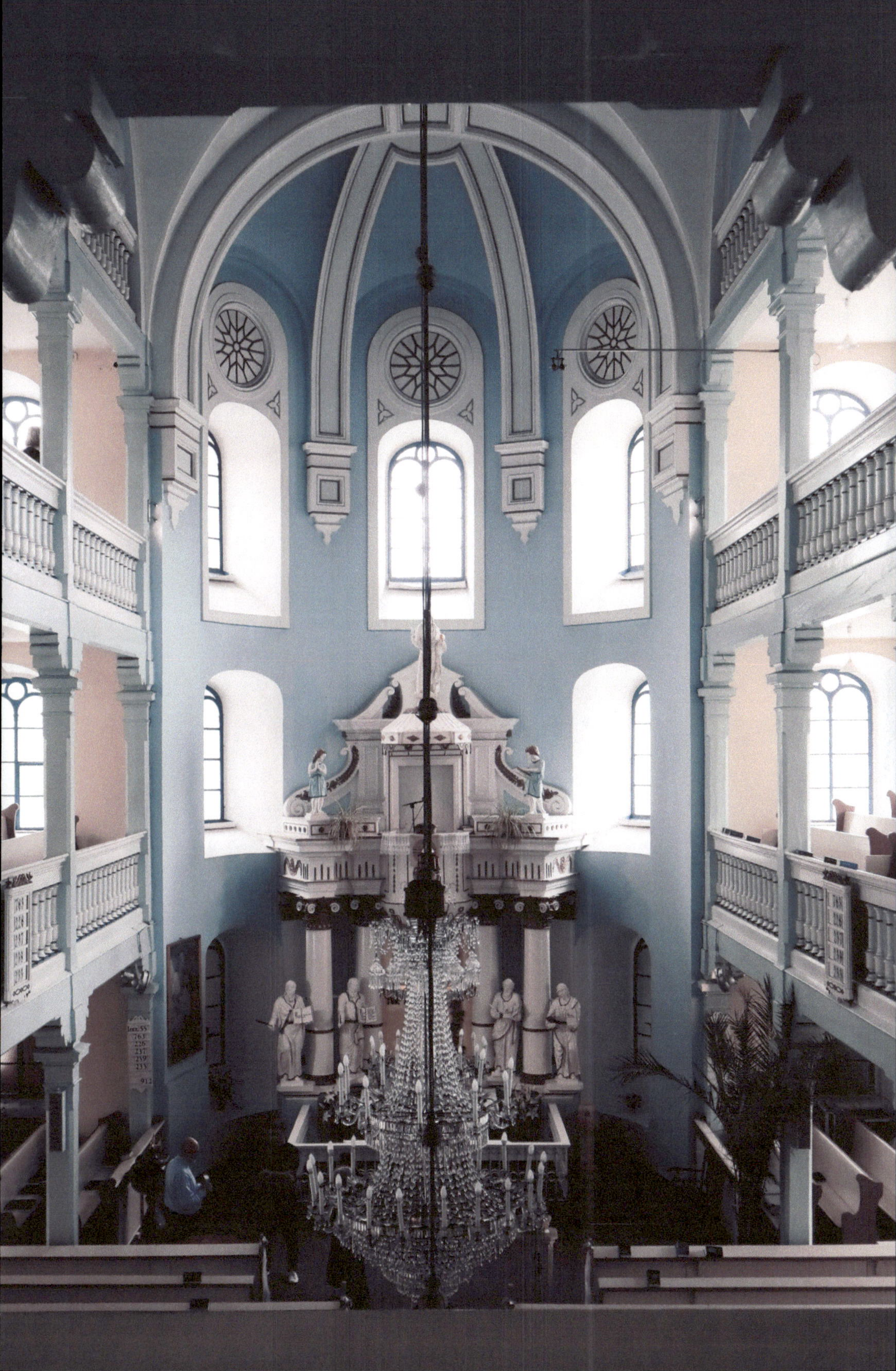

$\mathcal{Y}$our word is a lamp

to my feet and a light

to my path.

$\mathcal{P}$salm 119:105

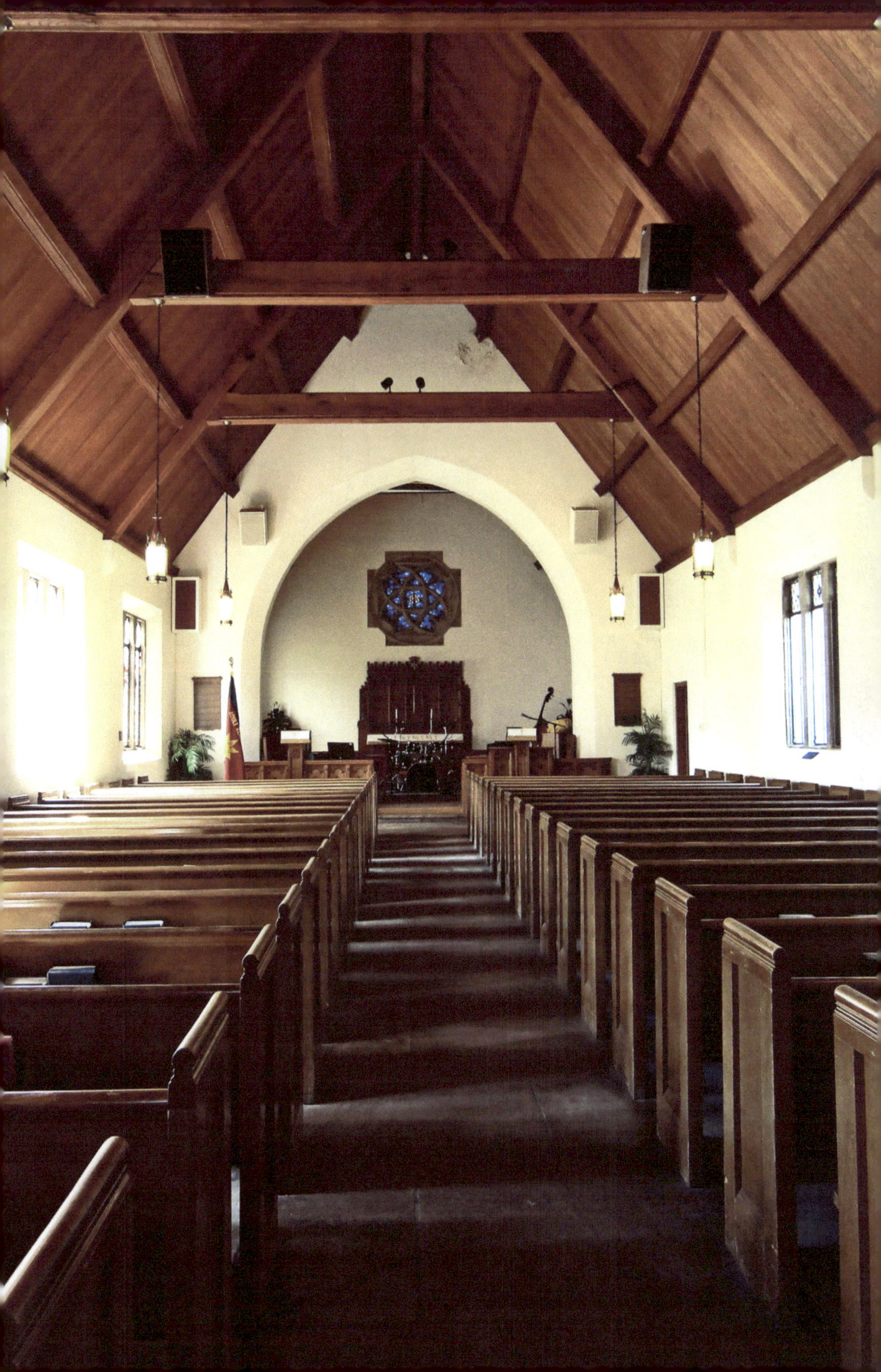

The Lord is my rock, my

fortress and my deliverer.

Psalm 18:2

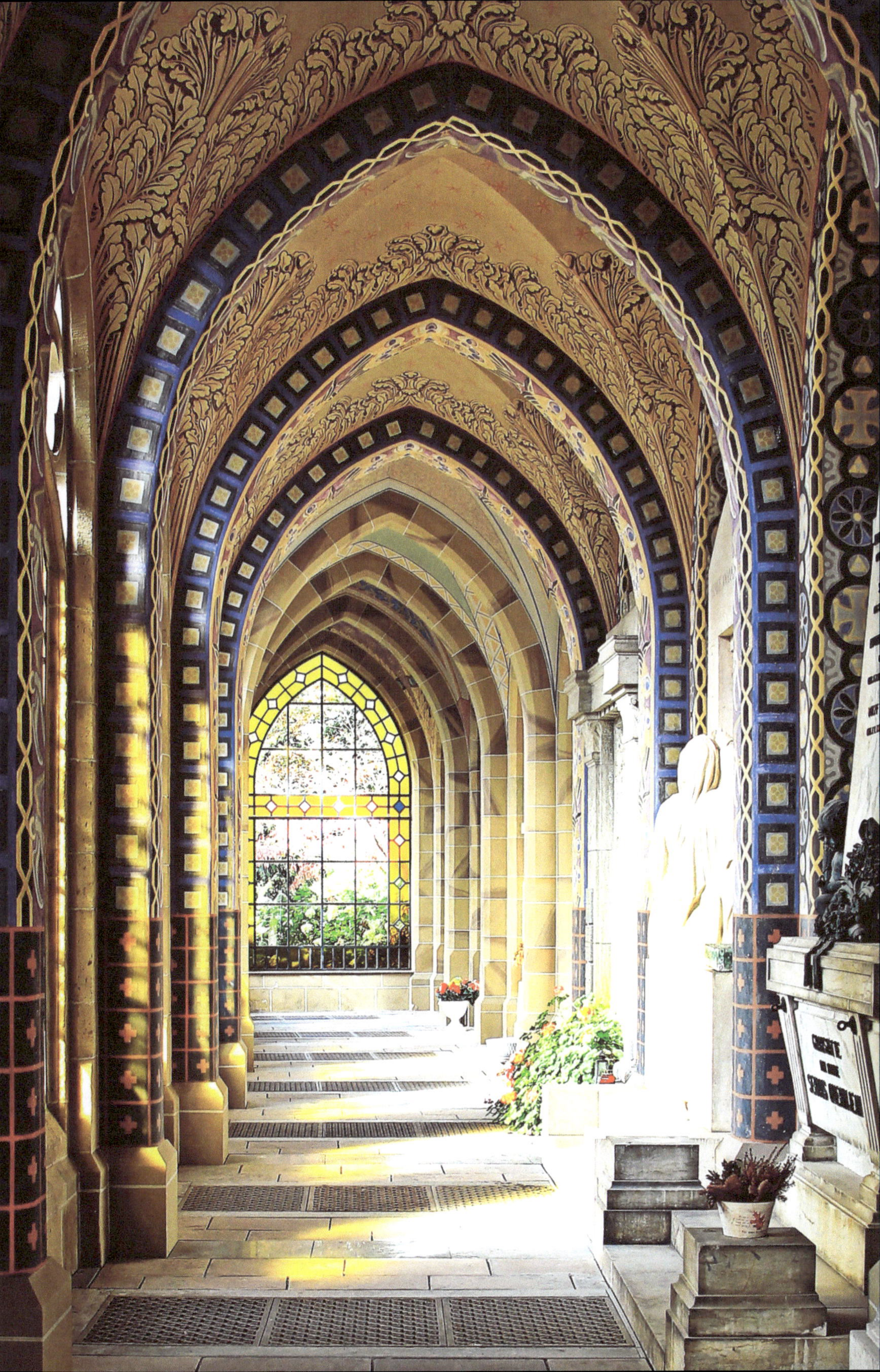

May your unfailing

love be with us, Lord,

even as we put our

hope in you.

Psalm 33:22

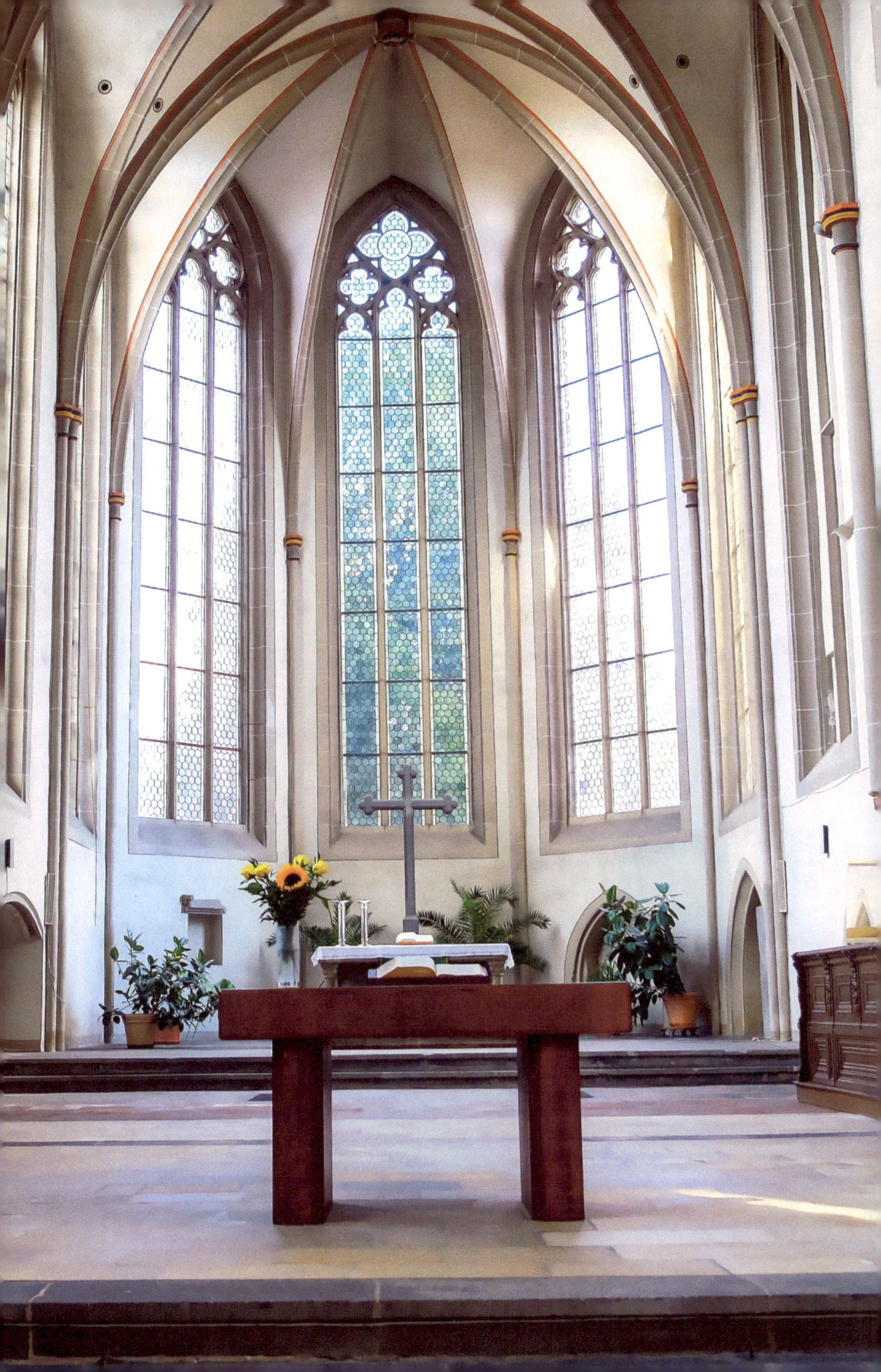

The heavens declare

the glory of God; the

skies proclaim the work

of his hands.

Psalm 19:1

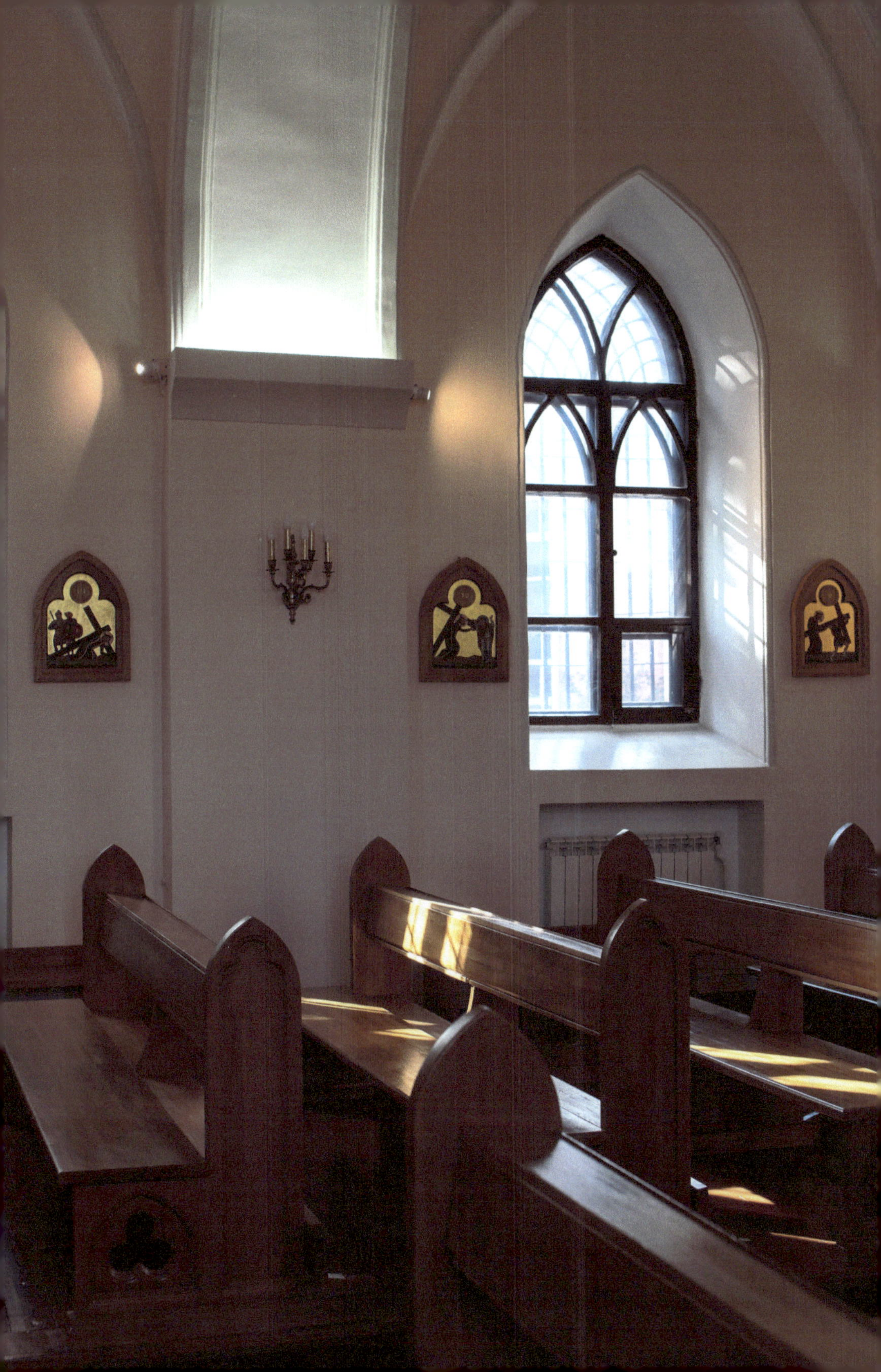

Give thanks to the Lord,

for he is good. His love

endures forever.

Psalm 107:1

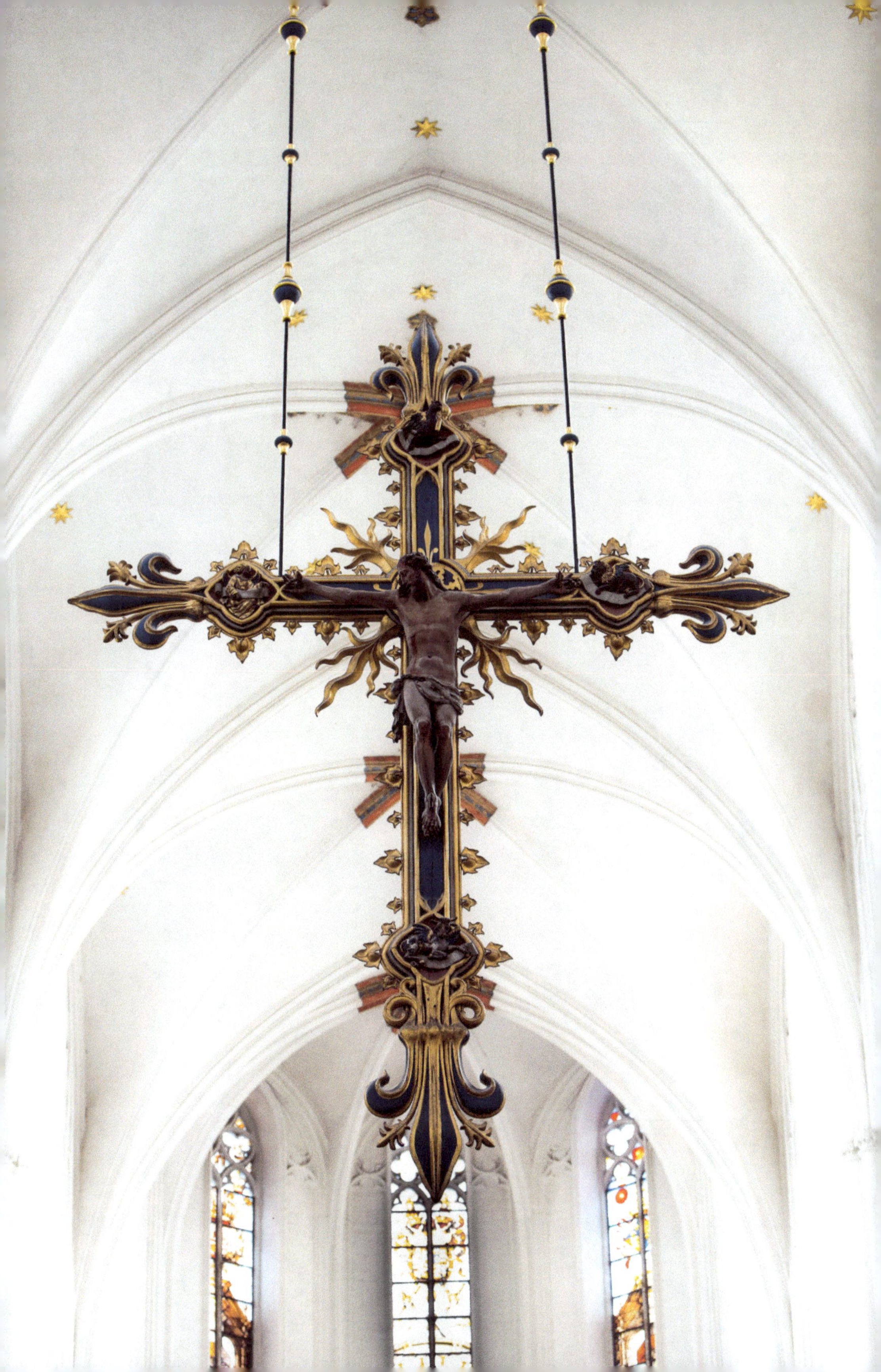

The Lord will watch over

your coming and going

both now and forever.

Psalm 121:8

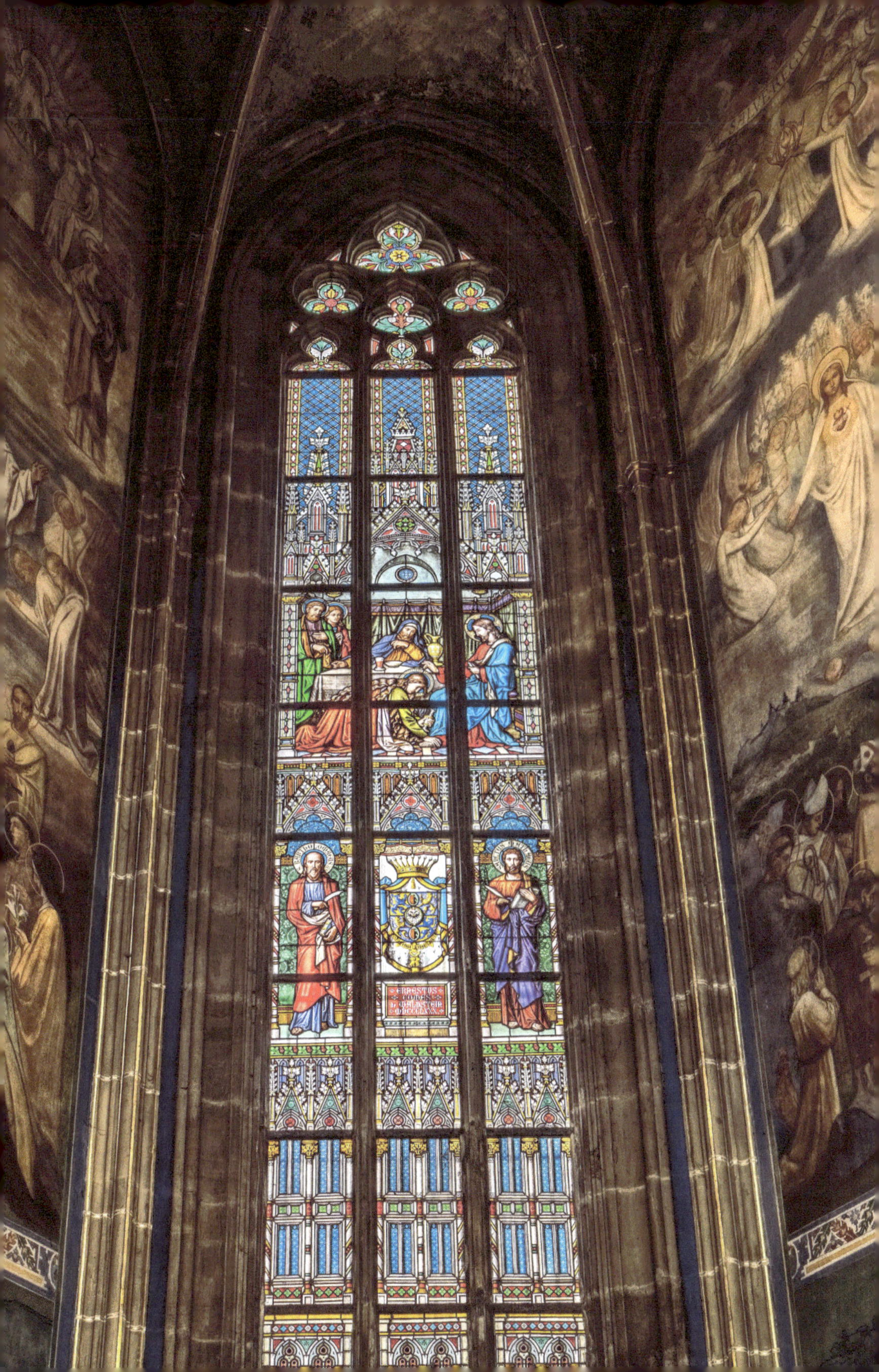

*T*he Lord is my shepherd,

I shall not want.

*P*salm 23:1

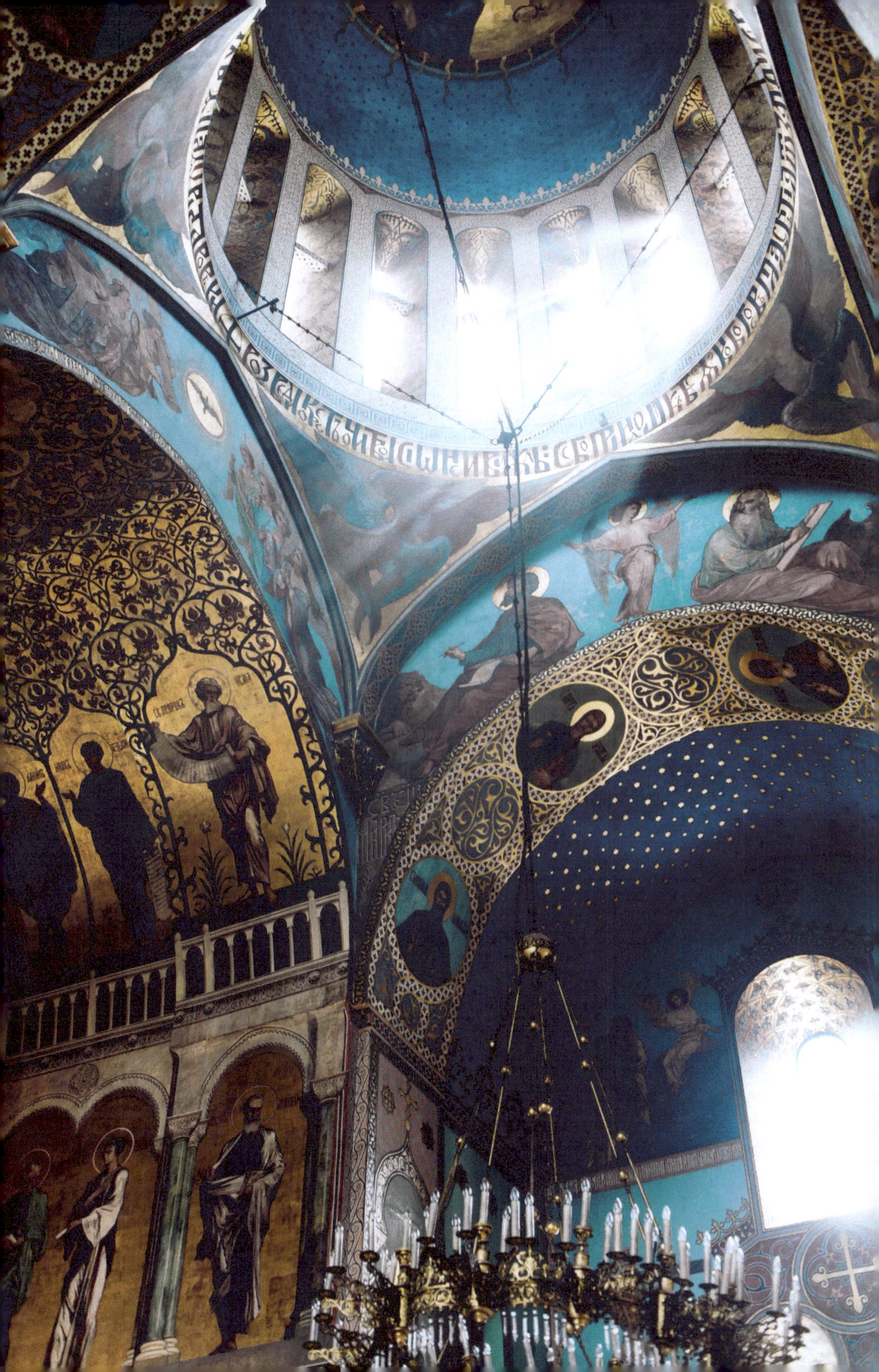

I sought the Lord, and

he answered me; he

delivered me from all

my fears.

Psalm 34:4

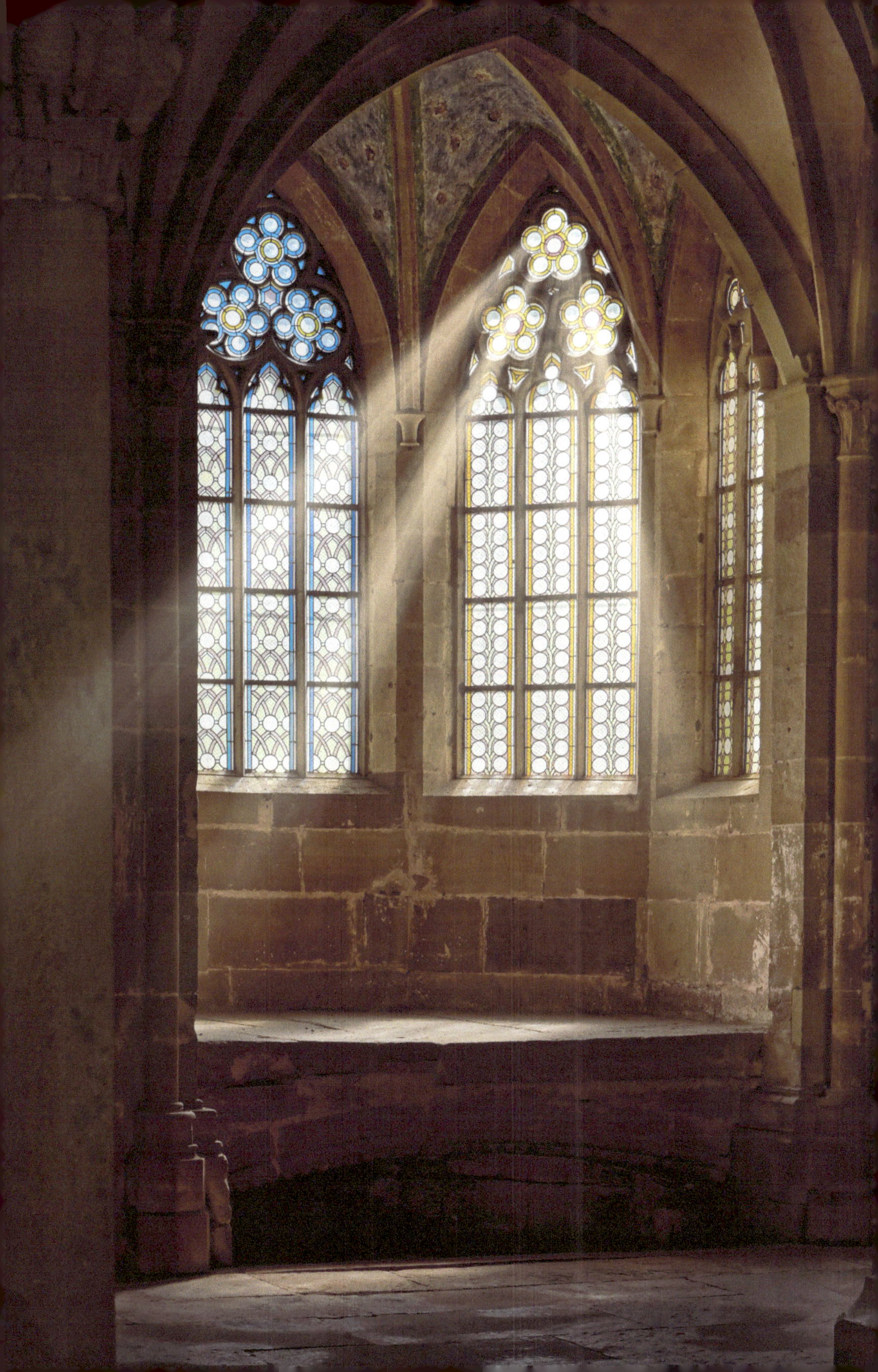

Cast your cares on

the Lord and he will

sustain you.

Psalm 55:22

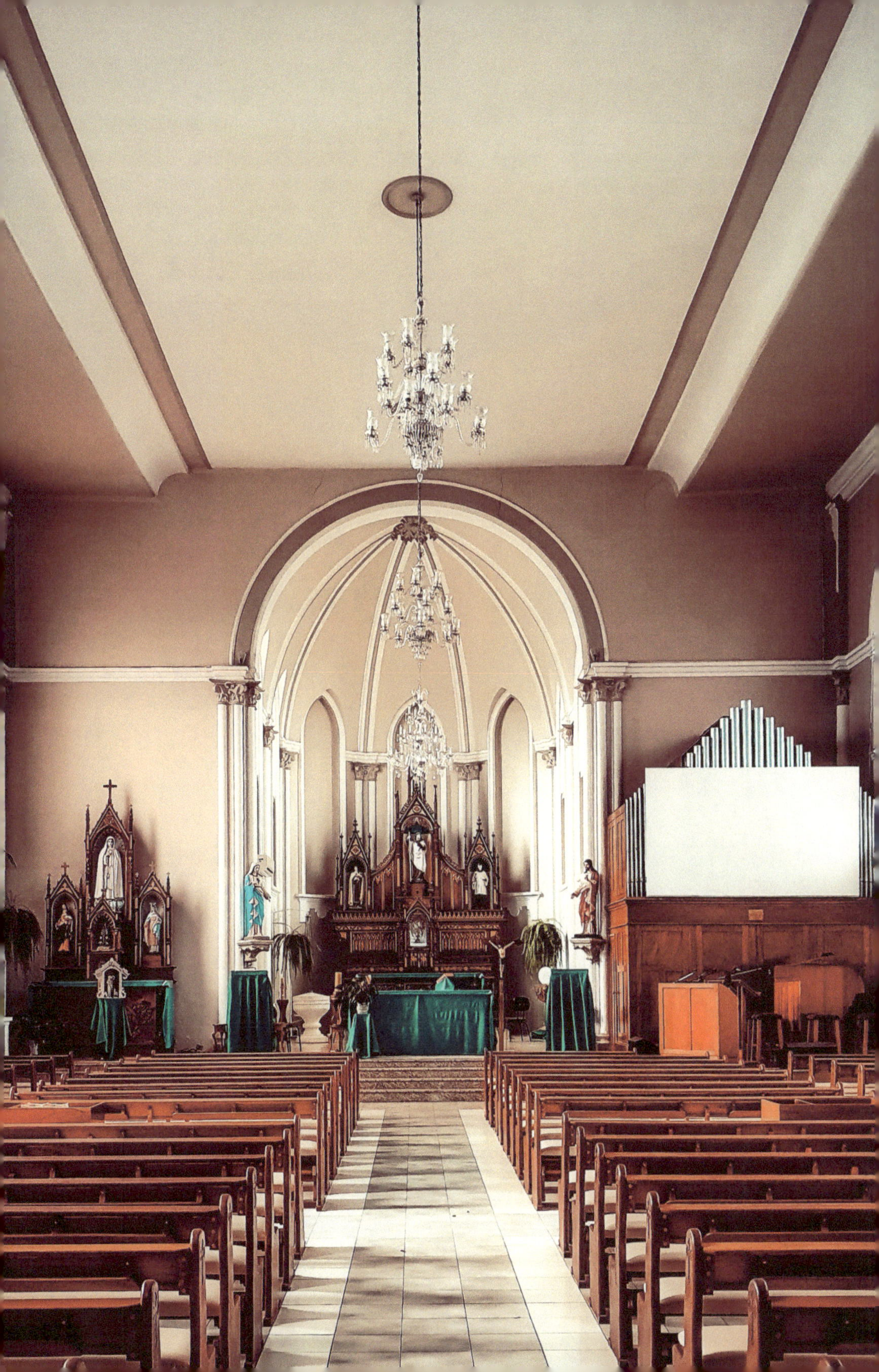

I will be glad and rejoice

in you; I will sing the

praises of your name.

Psalm 31:7

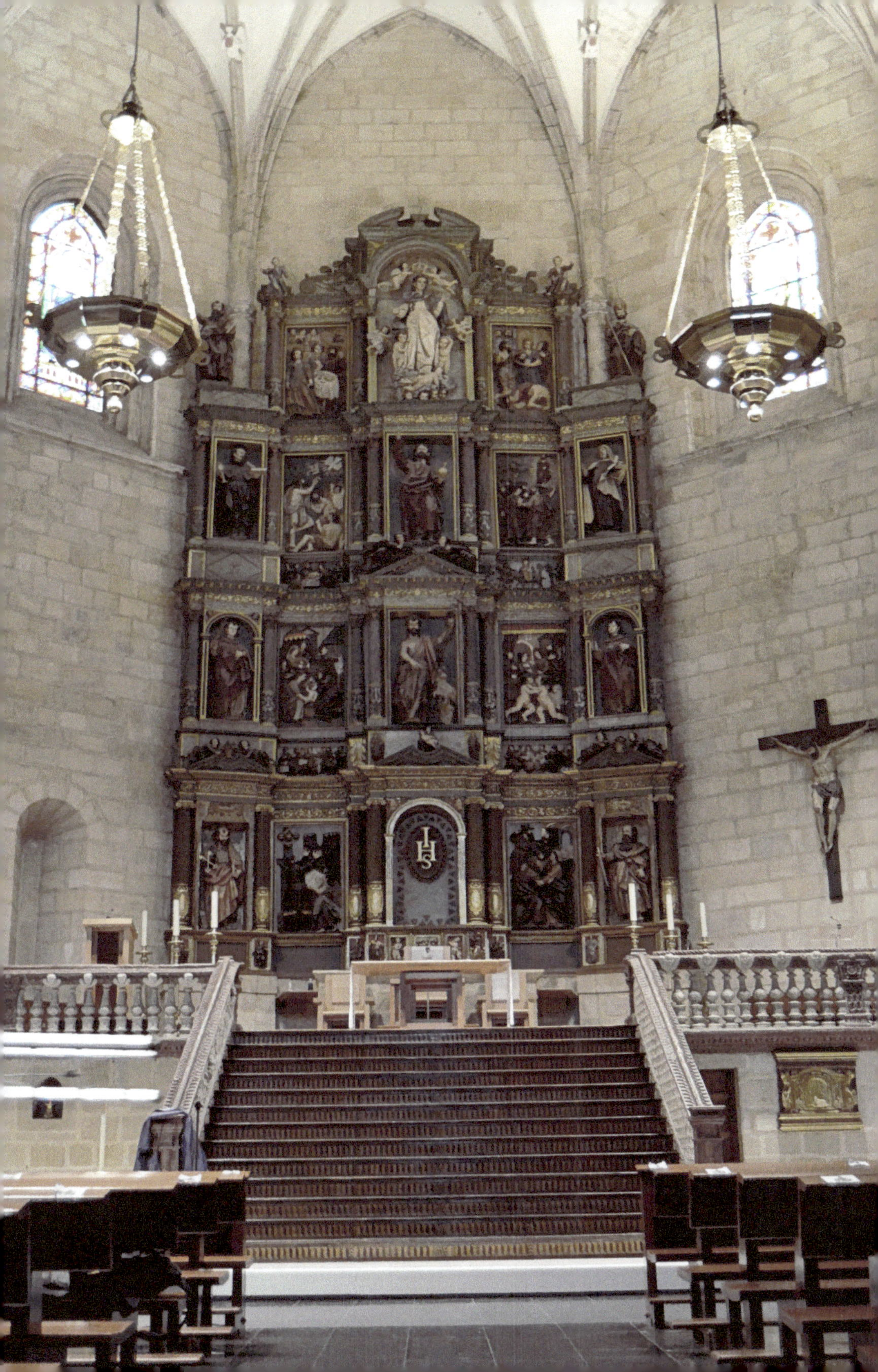

The Lord gives

strength to his people;

the Lord blesses his

people with peace.

Psalm 29:11

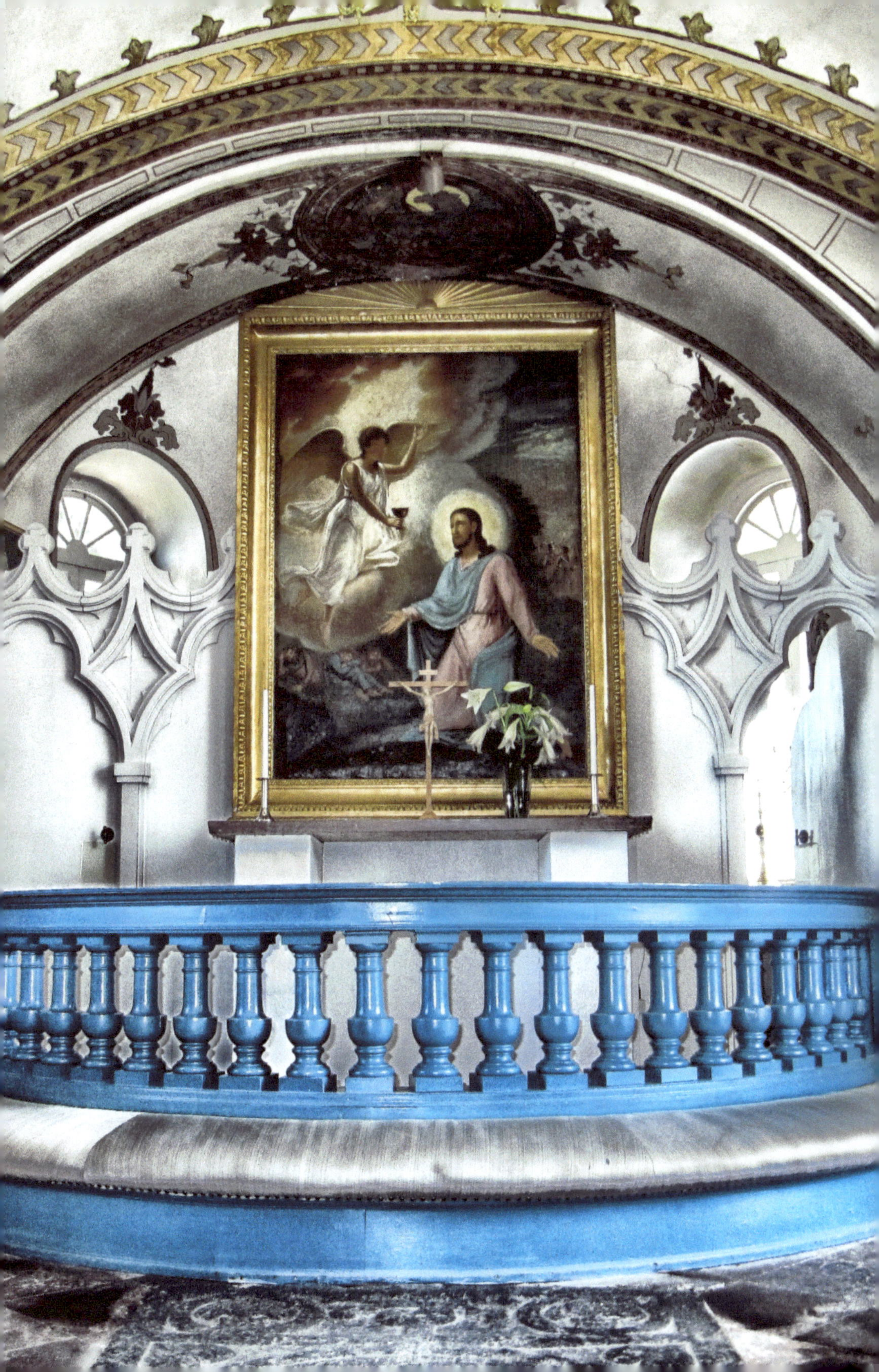

www.ingramcontent.com/pod-product-compliance
Lightning Source LLC
Chambersburg PA
CBHW041808260726
48664CB00036B/1479